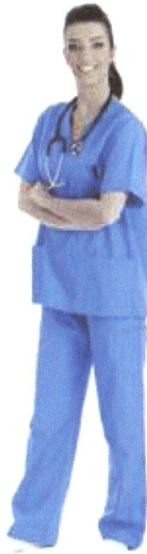

100 WAYS TO BE A NURSE AND LOVE IT (A Guide to Career Options and Choices in Nursing)

by Sherry Ronke

Get All The Books In The Series:

Table of Contents

1. CONTENT

INTRODUCTION

LIST OF CAREER OPTIONS FOR NURSES

Acting
Administration
Adult day care program
Ambulatory surgery
Anesthesia Nursing
Apheresis Nursing
Audiology
Auditors
Behavioral Health
Billing and coding.
Business Executives / Entrepreneur
Cardiology
Case Management
Clinical Instruction
Clinical Nurse Specialist Clinics
Community Educator
Consulting
Correctional
Cosmetology (Beauty Nurse)
Counseling Nurse
Critical Care
Dermatology
Dental
Dialysis

Doctor's office
Ear, Nose & Throat
Educator
Emergency
Fertility (reproductive nursing)
Fire Department
Flight Nursing
Forensic
Gastroenterology
Gerontology
Health Services Policy and decision-making
HIV/AIDS care
Holistic
Home Health Services
Hospice
Humanitarian services
ICU (Intensive Care Units)
Independent Practice/Business & Enterprise
Infection Control
Informatics
Inspectors
Insurance
Intravenous Nurse
Laboratory
Labor & Delivery
Labor Union
Legal Nurse Consultant
Managed Care
Managerial
Marketing & Sales Rep
Mass Media
Maternal/Child Health
MDS Coordinator/PRI Assessor

Medical Malpractice investigator
Medical Nursing
Medical-Surgical Nursing
Medical Transcription
Midwifery
Military
MR/DD
Neonatal
Neurology
Nurse Practitioner
Nursing Home
Obstetrics
Occupational
Operating room
Ophthalmology
Oncology
Orthopedic
Parish
Pediatric Nursing
Pharmaceutical
Plastic Surgical Nursing
Politics
Psychiatric Nursing
Public Health Nursing
Quality Assurance/QI
Quality Management
Radiological Nursing
Recruitment Specialist
Rehabilitation
Research
Respiratory Nursing
Revenue Management
School Nursing

Seminar/Personal Development
Staff Development
Substance Abuse
Surgical Nursing
Teaching (Faculty)
Transplant care
Travel (mobile)
United Nation
Urology
Visiting Nursing
Wound Care Nurse Specialist

EARNINGS AND JOB OPPORTUNITIES

SOURCES OF ADDITIONAL INFORMATION

A LIST OF SOME ASSOCIATIONS, WEB SITES &
RESOURCES

2. INTRODUCTION.

The inspiration to write this book came when I was in school for my Baccalaureate (BSN) program. I was thinking about what to do on completion of the program. I was already a Registered Nurse (RN) working in Home Health services. I have had some experience in medical-surgical (med-surg), outpatient clinic, and others. I was still ruminating on which type of Nursing I would like to go into. I said to myself, "let me just list the areas in which I have worked and then add other areas that I know so that I can choose". To my amazement, I easily wrote down 10, then 20, 30 and the list was growing. I never knew there could be so many career choices and options in Nursing. Therefore, I thought of how many of the more than four million nurses out there who were not aware of the choices they could make as they continue to grow in their career. So, this book was born.

As a nurse, when you have the information in this book, you do not have to feel burned out in any area of Nursing. You can always make a change. You have plenty of options. This book is for Registered Nurses (RN) and Licensed Practical Nurse (LPN), and people considering a career change to Nursing, as well as High school students who will like to begin a career in Nursing. The message is the same; you have so much room to grow and so many options from which to choose. It is my hope that you will find the information in this book helpful. Whatever is your reason for desiring to read this book, I hope you find it helpful. If you are aspiring to become a nurse, I believe that you need to have a caring heart because nursing is about caring.

Quite a lot of people say that they like Nursing but do not like the hospital or that they do not like the idea of being a bedside Nurse. Well, if you are someone like that, you do not have to remain in bedside forever. You can always choose from other areas. If you are considering a career in Nursing and you do not like the hospital or the bedside, you still have other choices. Although I must say that working at the bedside is a noble thing to do because you get a wonderful opportunity to demonstrate your caring heart in a practical way.

For every area of specialty described, it is required for you to be a trained Nurse. In addition to the basic general nursing training, specialty training is required which may range from one day to months or even years. If you are not already a nurse, you may seek admission to college, there are 2-year programs and there are four-year programs. There are three-year diploma programs mostly outside U.S. You may even start as a practical nurse, become a Licensed Practical Nurse or Licensed vocational Nurse, which is a one-year program, and grow from there.

3. NURSING OPTION AND CHOICES

ACTING

The Nurse can choose acting as a career. He/she plays the role of a nurse in drama, movies etc, and as a screenwriter, or scriptwriter.

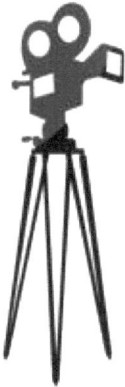

ADMINISTRATION

The Nurse specializes in administering the hospitals, sub-units in the hospital, the clinic etc. This is a leadership position.

ADULT DAY CARE PROGRAM

The Nurse works in the day care centers for adults. Mostly the participants at these centers are elderly, weak and cannot be alone at home when families are off to work. Sometimes the participants go for companionship.

AMBULATORY SURGERY
The nurse works in a setting in which patients undergo Day Surgery. The nurse prepares patients for the surgery, sends them to the operating room, receives them back from surgery, cares for them until the effect of anesthesia completely wears off and the clinical condition permits the patient to leave. Many places open only on weekdays. So, if you like weekends off, you may consider this option.

ANESTHESIA NURSE
The Nurse administers anesthesia during surgery, monitors the patient during and after surgery until the patient regains consciousness. This is an advanced position.

APHERESIS NURSING
The Nurse is involved in the process of collecting and harvesting blood, and the blood is, therapeutically separated, depending on the need, e.g. stem cell, platelets etc.

AUDIOLOGY
The Nurse trains as an audiologist. She makes use of a special equipment to test for hearing in pediatrics and adult, and works with patient on getting hearing aids.

AUDITORS
The Nurse works with health institutions to make sure that patient/ client's records are in accord with the regulations of accrediting bodies.

BEHAVIORAL HEALTH
The Nurse is a specialist in emotional health & wellness, helping clients to stay balanced at home and on the job. The Nurse works with the client to make living and working well possible. The nurse provides care as coach, advocate, and connects clients with assistance for everything, from childcare resource to treatment for depression, anxiety etc, and as a behavioral health nurse helps to improve health care outcomes for individual & families, fighting morbid behavior (e.g. phobias, anorexia, bulimia, substance abuse, obesity etc) needing counsel or seeking other support with life's challenges.

BILLING & CODING
The Nurse works to bill the insurance companies, Medicare and Medicaid and other third party payor system. This service is available in health institutions and other

private MD offices and home care. The nurse can work from home.

BUSINESS MANAGERS AND EXECUTIVES / ENTREPRENEUR

The nurse work to set up business entities and entrepreneurship in health care related field. Areas such as building, and running Nursing Homes, behavioral health homes and clinics, Medical Equipment sales and Supplies, Home health care agency, Health Care Staffing Agency and so many others.

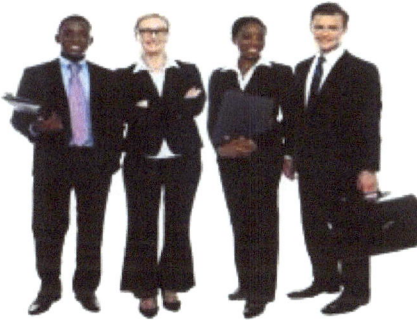

CARDIOLOGY

The Nurse specializes in the care of patients with heart problems. It could either be in the cardiac units inside the hospital, in the clinics.

CASE MANAGEMENT

The Nurse trains in case management to perform assessment plan and manage patient services and care, conduct research, analyze data. The aim is to promote quality, cost effective health care and human services for patient and their families.

CLINICAL INSTRUCTOR

The Nurse teaches student nurses in the hospital units. The clinical Instructor teaches the students the practical aspects of what they learn in the classroom. The nurse can also teach the Nurse Assistants or the Practical Nurse and in some cases other Professional Nurses.

CLINICAL NURSE SPECIALIST

The Nurse specializes in a specific area of nursing or subject area and He/she teaches other nurses that work in the area. Areas of specialty include pediatrics, geriatrics, and disability.

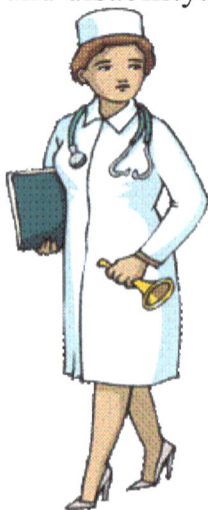

CLINICS

The Nurse works in clinics such as, outpatient clinics, or satellite clinics connected with the hospitals. A lot of time, the clinics are open Monday through Friday, and close on the weekends. Therefore, if you like to be off on the weekends, you may want to consider this option.

COMMUNITY EDUCATOR

The Nurse works mostly in Home care, acting as the liaison between the institution and the community and recruiting patients/clients for the facilities.

CONSULTING

The Nurse works as an independent Contractor in consultancy services, (e.g. educational consulting), in areas such as the establishment of new health care institutions or staffing agencies.

CORRECTIONAL

The Nurse works in the hospital and clinic of correctional facilities or the prison services.

COSMETOLOGY (BEAUTY NURSE)

The Nurse specializes in the art of permanent/non-permanent cosmetics. Cosmetology closely relates to plastic surgery, and the procedure could be invasive or non-invasive.

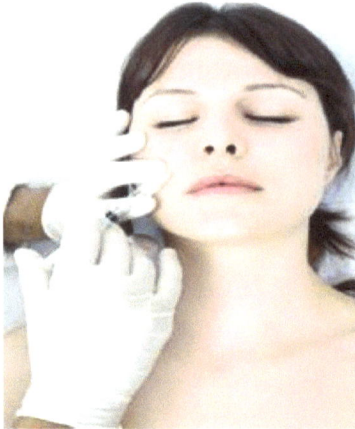

COUNSELING NURSE
There are different areas of counseling e.g. teenage pregnancy, sexual assault, substance abuse, child abuse etc. This service also extends to children and adults with physical, sensory and learning disabilities. The counseling nurse provides ongoing support to client and families. The nurse is a member of Early Intervention service and liaises with all agencies involved, both statutory and voluntary. The objective is to enhance the quality of life.

CRITICAL CARE
The Nurse ensures that critically ill patients and their families receive optimal care. Critically ill patients are the ones who are at high risk for actual or potential life

threatening health problems. The nurse works in, the intensive care unit, step down or transitional care units, emergency care departments, or post operative recovery.

DERMATOLOGY
The Nurse specializes in the care of patients with skin and hair problems. He/she works in the clinic or hospital units.

DENTAL
The Nurse cares for people with dental problems, including mouth surgery. They can work in the clinic, in the hospital units, or dental offices.

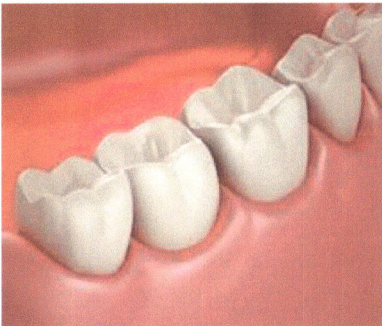

DIALYSIS
The Nurse works in hemo dialysis (artificial kidney) units, which could be in-patient or outpatient. The Nurse could also perform peritoneal dialysis.

DOCTOR'S OFFICE

The Nurse works in Doctor's private office, performing office and telephone triage, in addition to facilitating consultation with the Doctor during the patients' office visits. Many Doctors' offices are open only on weekdays.

EAR, NOSE & THROAT

The Nurse specializes in caring for patients with ear, nose and throat including surgeries in the said area.

EDUCATOR (Nurse)

The Nurse teaches in clinics, hospital units etc. She specializes in a particular subject area such as diabetes, sexually transmitted diseases, or abuse. So whenever there is a need for teaching patients in the subject area, the nurse is does so.

EMERGENCY

The Nurse works in the emergency room and with the ambulance,
specializing in emergency care and First Aid.

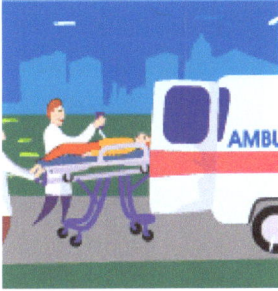

FERTILITY (Reproductive Nursing)

The Nurse works in infertility clinics, and specializes in-vitro fertilization. The core practice is Assisted Reproduction Technology: the Nurse works in clinics that offer treatments such as correction of hormonal problems, or facilitation of matches between egg donors and their recipients, and in counseling program to help couples cope with emotional issues relating to infertility.

FIRE DEPARTMENT

The nurse could work in the fire department to work as a part of the emergency crew, during fire outbreak or any kind of emergency.

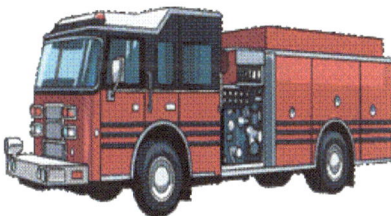

FLIGHT NURSING
The Nurse is involved in the emergency medical response by air. It is like Air ambulance. There are subspecialties also, e.g. pediatric team, neonatal, general transport team, and high-risk obstetrics. Employment opportunities are available in the private sector, government and military.

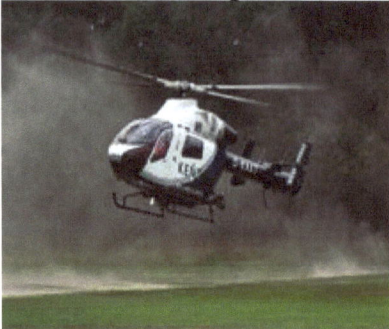

FORENSIC
The Nurse works with law enforcement to investigate crimes – analyze crime-related samples in the forensic labs and may care for crime victims.

GASTROENTEROLOGY
The Nurse specializes in the care of patient with stomach and intestinal problems at the in-patient care level or investigational units such as x-ray with barium, viewing the tract as in endoscopies etc.

GERONTOLOGY NURSE

The Nurse specializes in the care of the elderly, and may become a Geriatric nurse practitioner. (See Nurse Practitioner)

GYNECOLOGICAL NURSE

The Nurse specializes in working with patients with gynecological problems.

HEALTH SERVICES POLICY AND DECISION MAKING

The Nurse is involved in decision-making and in enacting rules that govern the day-to-day running of the institution where he or she works. Professional Nursing Organizations promote and advocate the participation of nursing in local, national and international health decision-making and policy development bodies, and committees. Nurses that work in this area could work as lobby groups to persuade lawmakers. They sometimes participate in politics.

HIV/AIDS CARE

The Nurse specializes in HIV/AIDS care, research, prevention and policy.

HOLISTIC
The Nurse works as a practitioner that cares for patients, spirit, soul and body. The Nurse views the patient as a whole because of the belief that issues in patient's lives are interrelated. This is where the Alternative Practitioners come in.

HOME HEALTH SERVICES
Home Health Services, is a big area. Some of the several options from which to choose are; the visiting nurse, coordinators, and intake nurse.

HOSPICE
The Nurse cares for the dying, the terminally ill in hospice facility or in the comfort of the patients home. The Nurse also counsels and supports the patients and their families.

HUMANITARIAN SERVICES
An example is the Red Cross society. They respond to human health needs during natural or man-made (e.g. wars) disasters. It involves traveling. Many private not-for-profit organizations perform this type of service and Nurses play vital roles in caring for human victims.

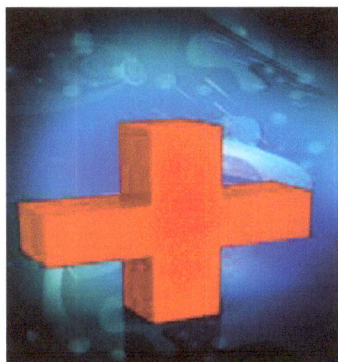

ICU (INTENSIVE CARE UNIT). See critical care

INDEPENDENT PRACTICE /BUSINESS & ENTERPRISE

The nurses may establish business enterprises, mostly in health related areas such as Nursing Agency (providing Nurses to Hosp/Nursing Homes on per diem bases), medical supplies company, health Journal, uniforms and others. The nurse becomes an employer of labor.

INFECTION CONTROL

The Nurse works as the Infection Control Nurse within the hospital, collecting data from each unit regarding any occurrence of infection. Other responsibilities are to monitor compliance with rules and regulations and policy relating to infection control. The Nurse also teaches members of staff about the measures of reducing the spread of infection

INFORMATIC (NURSING INFORMATICS)

The Nurse works with (computer) clinical information systems, educational appliances, data collection/ research application, and administrative decision support systems.

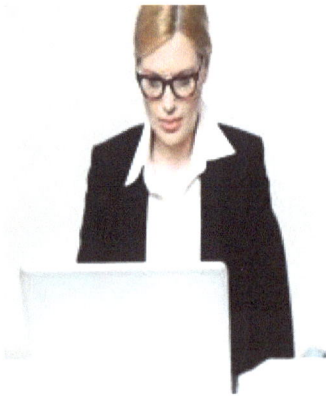

INSPECTORS (NURSE INSPECTORS)

They work with the accrediting bodies/insurance. They visit health institutions and check patients' chart in compliance with rules and regulations.

INSURANCE

The Nurse works with the Health insurance companies to approve services that patients utilize to make sure the services requested are needed and necessary.

INTRAVENOUS NURSE

The Nurse specializes in intravenous methods of treating patient, as in performing PICC lines, administration of meds, ports etc.

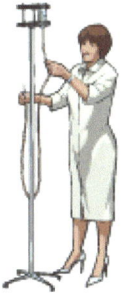

LABORATORY

The Nurse works in the lab. Sometimes it depends on the policy of the hospital. The nurse may collect specimen, store them, take blood etc.

LABOR UNION

The Nurse runs Nurses' labor union and helps to organize new ones, to see to the welfare of members.

LEGAL NURSE CONSULTANT

A legal Nurse Consultant is a registered nurse who has acquired legal skills to handle personal injury and medical malpractice litigation. Job opportunities are available in law firms, insurance companies, legal department of health related corporations and government agencies.

MANAGED CARE
The Nurse works with the managed care - Health Insurance Company to make sure that health Care institution does not provide unnecessary service for their clients. This is to avoid paying too much money as reimbursement.

MANAGERIAL
The Nurse manages other nurses. This is a leadership position. Managers manage sub units in many hospitals.

MARKETING AND SALES REPRESENTATIVE
The Nurse may work for pharmaceutical and medical supplies companies to market their products to clients such as healthcare institutions, and professionals. It involves traveling in many cases. If you love traveling, this may be for you.

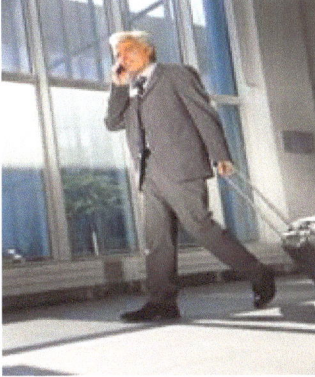

MASS MEDIA
The Nurse works in mass media as a reporter, adviser, producer etc on health related issues with newspapers, magazines, radio, television etc.

MATERNAL/CHILD
The Nurse specializes in caring for the patient during pregnancy (mother and baby) and, after delivery.

MDS COORDINATOR/PRI ASSESOR
The Nurse specializes in MDS and PRI, which are instruments used by Medicare and Medicaid for reimbursement purpose to health care providers or Institutions.

MEDICAL MALPRACTICE INVESTIGATOR

The nurse specializes in investigating any type of malpractice, works mostly with insurance company and government, and reviews patients' charts and conduct interviews with the people involved.

MEDICAL NURSING

The Nurse works in general acute/chronic illness units where they care for patients with all manners of sickness. In some hospitals, this unit/area joins the surgical unit, so the nurse performs as both medical nurse and surgical nurse.

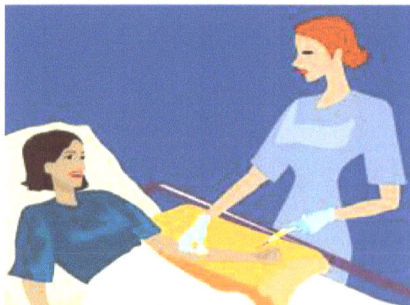

MEDICAL-SURGICAL, NURSING (MED-SURG)

Many believe that medical-surgical nursing is the bedrock of any type of Nursing. It is widely known (and strongly recommended) that you should have at least one year experience in this type of nursing to serve as your foundation in nursing career. Med-Surg Nurse performs the traditional role of bedside nursing, caring for the sick in the medical/surgical units in the hospital. Usually, it is general acute sickness such as infection malaise.

Sometimes the unit splits into medical or surgical units or could be together especially in smaller hospital. In the surgical units, the nurse cares for people who are going for surgery or are recovering from surgeries.

MEDICAL TRANSCRIPTION
The nurse works as a Medical Transcriptionist, recording conversations and procedures during consultation, surgeries or meeting by the Doctors, Surgeons, or managers and administrators, and later transcribing such conversation into readable version.

MIDWIFERY
The Midwife is independent in some places. She cares for the pregnant mother throughout pregnancy and delivery. Some patients prefer a midwife to monitor them during pregnancy and delivery especially for religious reasons.

MILITARY
The Nurse joins any arm of the military - the Army, the Navy and the Air Force or the Marines - to care for sick military personnel. Some receive military training while some work as civilians in military hospitals.

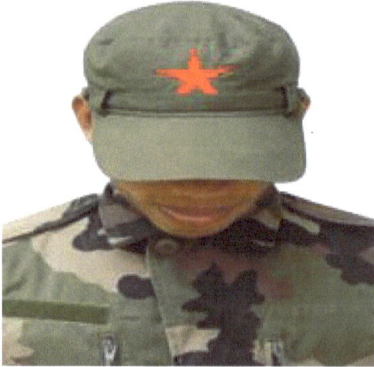

MR/DD

The Nurse specializes in working with the mentally retarded and clients with developmental disabilities.

NEONATAL

A neonate is a newborn up to 28 days after birth. The neonatal nurse specializes in taking care of the new born, infants and their families.

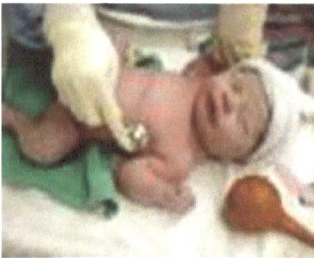

NEUROLOGY

The Nurse specializes in the care of patients with neurological problems. That is clients with nervous system dysfunction such as stoke, brain and spinal cord cancer, back injury and epilepsy. Job areas include ICU, in-patients, clinics, homes, and hospice.

NURSE PRACTITIONER
The Nurse practitioner is a registered nurse who has a master degree in nurse practitioner. This field is further divided to subspecialty like family nurse practitioner, pediatrics etc. The nurse practitioner has some degree of independence - able to prescribe some medications, performs physical examination and consultation service.

NURSING HOME
The Nurse works in the residence facility most of the time, for the elderly with chronic or sub acute medical problems. The nursing home patients virtually live there. They are there for months or years and a lot of time for the rest of their lives.

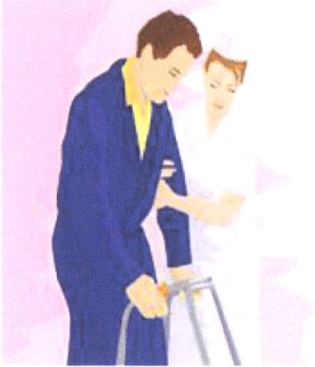

OBSTETRICS

The Nurse specializes in the care of patient during pregnancy, labor and delivery. Experience in Newborn care is necessary.

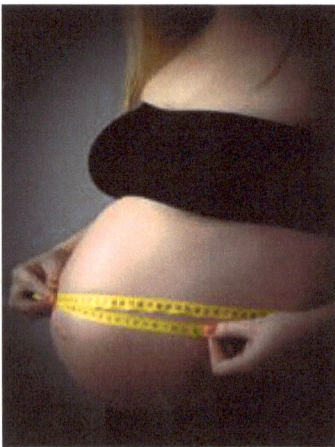

OCCUPATIONAL

The Nurse works in the clinic or health centers of companies, factories, staff health services within the hospitals or any institution for that matter. A lot of time, they work Monday through Friday.

OPERATING ROOM
The Nurse who specializes in OR (operating room) cares for the patient during surgery, works with the surgeon for the success of the surgery and is responsible for the smooth running of the operating theatre, the instruments and medications.

OPHTALMOLOGY
The nurse specializes in full range of ophthalmic and optical services.

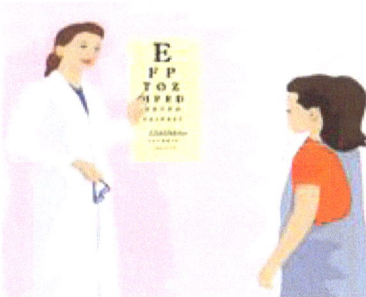

ONCOLOGY
The Nurse cares for people with cancer diagnosis. It could be a unit in the hospital or part of the medical-surgical unit. Such nurse may deal with various forms of cancer. In some other cases, there are many subspecialties with each based on a type of cancer.

ORTHOPEDIC

The Nurse works in areas that specialize in the care of skeletal disorders (bone problems), and can work in the orthopedic clinics.

PARISH

This is a type of nursing within a religious organization or community, in which the nurse takes care of sick members needing help or reaches out to the community. Spiritual dimension is central to parish nursing practice. The mission is to integrate the practice of faith with the practice of nursing.

PEDIATRIC NURSING

This is the Nursing Care of children. It may be subdivided into med-surg., pediatric surgery, pediatric clinic, pediatric intensive care and many others. You may specialize in your area of interest while you attend to children only.

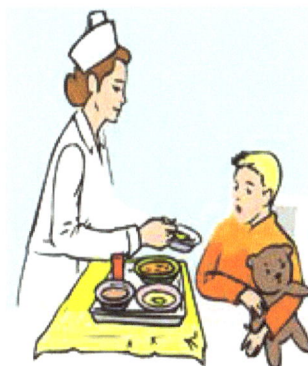

PHARMACEUTICAL
The Nurse works in the pharmaceutical company as a Research Nurse or as a Sales Representative. The sales part involves traveling.

PLASTIC SURGERY NURSING
The Nurse specializes in plastic and reconstructive surgery either for cosmetic purpose or as a form of treatment, e.g. hair transplant and nose job.

POLITICS
The Nurse gets involved in lobbying against political decision that may adversely affect nursing practice or Nursing profession. The nurse works closely with the unions, and may sometimes be actively involved in the politics.

PSYCHIATRIC NURSING
The Nurse works in mental health area, mostly in the hospital or outpatient clinic or emergency room, also in home visits or mobile crisis team.

PUBLIC HEALTH NURSING
As a Public Health Nurse, you work with the local or municipal government and private agencies. The focus is preventive Health. You are involved in enhancing the health of the population.

QUALITY ASSURANCE/ QUALITY IMPROVEMENT
The Nurse works with regulatory bodies to ensure that health care institutions and agencies follow the prescribed standard of care.

QUALITY MANAGEMENT
The Nurse works as a quality manager who performs quality audits regularly in the nursing units, the aim of which is to ensure that nursing staff maintain a high standard of nursing care and service constantly.

RADIOLOGICAL NURSING
The Nurse takes care of patient undergoing some type of X-ray, MRI, Barium Enema/meal, Mammogram, and is

responsible for promoting excellence and continuity of patient care in diagnostic or therapeutic imaging.

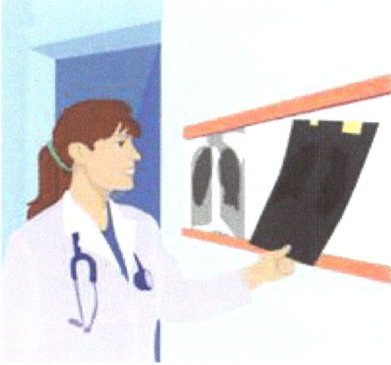

RECRUITMENT SPECIALIST
The Nurse is responsible for recruiting new nursing staff to the nursing department of the institutions and facilities.

REHABILITATION
The Nurse cares for patients who have some kind of structural damage. Such patients need to get back to their pre-damage condition or adjust to living within the limitation of disability.

RESEARCH
The Nurse works in the research field, testing new medications, types of treatments and their impacts on patients' condition and care.

RESPIRATORY NURSING
The Nurse works in the respiratory units, manages ventilators, chest clinics, chronic respiratory problems etc.

REVENUE MANAGEMENT
The Nurse works in the revenue management team, - jobs include how to handle budget allocated to Nursing in an institution, how to generate funds and how to manage funds effectively.

SCHOOL NURSE
The Nurse works in schools from elementary even up to college level, performing various responsibilities depending on the level of school. Job may include keeping children health records, making sure their immunizations are up to date, serving as first aid provider and giving health talks on common health problems especially the preventable ones.

SEMINAR/PERSONAL DEVELOPMENT
The Nurse teaches or organizes seminars on personal and professional development in (classes and conferences) either as an employee or as an employer.

STAFF DEVELOPMENT

The Nurse works in the education department of the hospital or Nursing Home as the in-service training nurse. There are mandatory classes stipulated by law. Also members of staff need new information, and trends that will help them to best perform their jobs.

SUBSTANCE ABUSE

The Nurse could walk with people (client) who are on substance use. It could be in the in-patient or outpatient.

SURGICAL NURSING

The nurse cares for people who have had one surgery or another. The department could be broken into specialties depending on the type of surgery: For example, orthopedic surgery, cardiac (heart), gastrointestinal surgery or pediatric surgery.

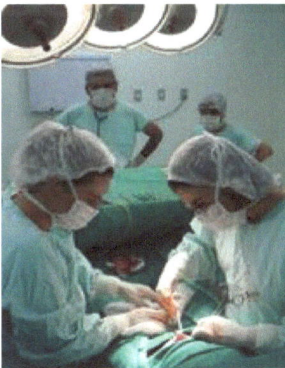

TEACHING (FACULTY)

The Nurse lectures in the nursing program in colleges and schools, where professional nurses and practical/vocational nurses are trained.

TRANSPLANT CARE

The Nurse counsels and prepares the patient before, during and after transplant. Tissue transplant involves special care.

TRAVEL (MOBILE)

The Nurse works with staffing agencies that provide short-term assignments ranging from 2-13 weeks to institution all over the country. If you love traveling, this may be for you.

UNITED NATIONS

The Nurse may work with the United Nations to serve in different Nations.

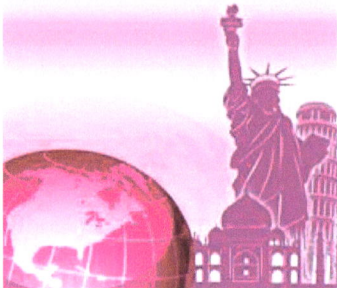

UROLOGY
The Nurse works in the unit that cares for patient with urinary tract problems including diagnostic procedures, surgery etc.

VISITING NURSE
The visiting nurse is part of the Home Health Services and the nurse visits from home to home, primarily to teach patients and to perform procedure that patients are unable to do. Where possible the nurse eventually teaches the patient/family how to perform such procedure e.g. injection administration, wound care etc.

WOUND CARE NURSE SPECIALIST
The Nurse trains in the treatment of wound/ulcer and provides consultation to other nurses on wound care.

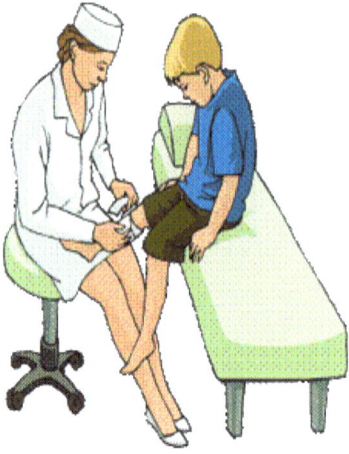

4. EARNINGS AND JOB OPPORTUNITIES

Job opportunities are great. According to the Department of Labor and Vital Statistics, "employment of Registered Nurses is expected to grow faster than the average for all occupation through 2012 and because the occupation is very LARGE many new jobs will result" Earnings: Median yearly salary is about $50,000 to $60,000.

Sources of Additional Information.
For information on a career as a registered nurse and nursing education, contact:
National League for Nursing, 61 Broadway, New York, NY10006
Internet: http://www.nln.org

For a list of BSN, graduate, and accelerated nursing programs, contact:
American Association of Colleges of Nursing, 1 Dupont Circle NW., Suite 530, Washington, DC 20036. Internet: http://www.aacn.nche.edu

Information of Registered Nurses also is available from: American Nurses Association, 600 Maryland Ave. SW., Washington, DC 20024-2571. Internet: http://www.nursingworld.org

5. NURSES ASSOCIATIONS AND RESOURCES

A LIST OF SOME ASSOCIATIONS, WEB SITES AND RESOURCES.

ACTING
Resource: movie industry
Web: www.scriptnurse.com

AMBULATORY SURGERY
Association: 1) Federated Ambulatory surgery Association
2) Day Surgery Association
3) American Academy of Ambulatory care nursing
Web: www.fasa.org

ANESTHESIA NURSE
Association: American Association of Nurse Anesthetists
Web: www.anesthesis-nursing.com
www.aana.com

CARDIOLOGY
Association: 1) American Heart Society
2) Cardiological Nurse Association
Web: Cardiology Online

CASE MANAGEMENT
Association: Case Management Society of America

CLINICAL INSTRUCTION
Association: Oncology Nursing Society
Web: www.ons.org
CLINICAL NURSE SPECIALIST
Association: National Association of Clinical Nurse Specialist
Web: www.nacns.org

CLINICS
Association: Clinic & Office Nurses Association
Web: www.nurses.ab.ca

COUNSELING NURSE
Web: www.elsevier.com

DENTAL
Association: British Association of Dental Nurses
Web: www.badn.org

DIALYSIS
Association: 1) International Society of Peritoneal Dialysis
     2) Nephrology Nurses Association
Web: www.ispd.org

DOCTOR'S OFFICE
Association: Clinic & office Nurses Association
Web: www.nurses.ab.ca

EDUCATOR

Association: Member-American college of Nursing.
Web: Nurse Educators/Association.org

EMERGENCY
Association: Emergency Nurses Association
Web: www.ena.org

FLIGHT NURSING
Association: National Flight Nurse
Web: www.flightnursing.com

FORENSIC
Association: International Association of Forensic Nurses
Web: www.forensicnurse.org

HIV/AIDS CARE
Association: Association of Nurses in AIDS Care
Web: www.anacnet.org

HOLISTIC
Association: American Holistic Nurses Association
Web: www.ahna.org

HOME HEALTH SERVICES
Web: www.nahc.org

HUMANITARIAN SERVICES
Web: www.zimply.com
    www.redcross.com

INDEPENDENT PRACTICE/BUSINESS & ENTERPRISE
Association: National Association of Independent Nurses
Web: www.independentrn.com

INFECTION CONTROL
Association: Infection Control Nurses Association
Web: www.icna.com

INFORMATICS
Association: American Nursing Informatics Association
Web: www.ania.org

LEGAL NURSE CONSULTANT
Association: Association of Legal Nurse Consultants
Web: www.aalnc.org

MIDWIFERY
Association: Independent midwives
Web: www.independentmidwives.org

MILITARY
Web: www.Anzacsteel.com

NEONATAL
Association: National Association of Neonatal Nurses
Web: www.nann.org

NURSE PRACTITIONER
Association: 1) American College of Nurse Practitioners

2) American Academy of Nurse practitioner

Web: www.aanp

www.nurse.org

NEUROLOGY

Association: American Association of Neuroscience Nurse (AANN)

Web: www.aann.org

OCCUPATIONAL

Association: American Association of Occupational Health

Web: www.aaohn.org

OPERATING ROOM

Association: 1) The association of Peri-operative registered nurses

2) Operating Room Nurses Association

Web: www.ornac

AORN online

ORTHOPEDIC

Association: National Association of orthopedic nurses

Web: www.orthonurse.org

PARISH

Association: 1) Iowa Nurses Association/Parishing

2) Canadian Association for Parish nursing ministry

Web: www.capnm.ca

www.iowanurses.org/parish

PEDIATRIC NURSING

Association: Society for Pediatric Nurses

Web: www.pednurses.org/

PLASTIC SURGICAL NURSING
Association: American Society of plastic Surgery nurses
Web: www.aspsn.org

PSYCHIATRIC NURSING
Association: American Psychiatric Nurses Association
Web: www.apna.org

PUBLIC HEALTH NURSING
Association: American Public Health Association (APHA)
Web: www.publichealth.mechanicalcentral.org
     www.Publichealthnurse.org

RADIOLOGICAL NURSING
Association: Radiological Nurses Association
Web: www.arna.net

REHABILITATION
Association: Association of Rehabilitation
Web: www.rehabnurse.org

RESEARCH
Association: Clinical Research Nurse Association
Web: www.man.ac.uk

RESPIRATORY NURSING
Association: Association of Respiratory Nurse Specialist
Web: www.respiratorynursingsociety.org

SCHOOL NURSE
Association: National Association of School Nurses
Web: www.nasn.org

STAFF DEVELOPMENT
Association: National Nursing staff Development organization
Web: www.nnsdo.org

SURGICAL NURSING
Association: 1) American pediatric Nurse Association
         2) Association of Preoperative Registered Nurses
         3) American Society of Plastic Surgical Nurses
Web: AORN online

TEACHING(FACULTY)
Association: American Association of colleges of Nursing
Web: www.nursingfaculty.com

VISITING
SEE HOME HEALTH SERVICE

WOUND CARE NURSE SPECIALIST
Association: 1) American Professional wound care association
         2) The wound ostomy and conference nurses society
(WOCN)
Web: www.zimply.com
     www.aswcjournal.com

Career Options For Lawyers

Get All The Books In The Series:

CAREER OPTIONS FOR LAWYERS

Career Optios For Doctors

Career Options For Teachers and Educators

Career Options For Engineers

Career Options For Journalists

Career Options For Scientists.

The Fat Loss Factor

Professional and Technical books